# Microdosing & Growing Psilocybin Mushrooms

## A Beginner's 3-Week Step-by-Step Guide for PTSD Relief, Mood Stabilization, and Mental Well-Being

copyright © 2025 Felicity Paulman

All rights reserved No part of this book may be reproduced, or stored in a retrieval system, or transmitted in any form or by any means, electronic, mechanical, photocopying, recording, or otherwise, without express written permission of the publisher.

# Disclaimer

By reading this disclaimer, you are accepting the terms of the disclaimer in full. If you disagree with this disclaimer, please do not read the guide.

All of the content within this guide is provided for informational and educational purposes only, and should not be accepted as independent medical or other professional advice. The author is not a doctor, physician, nurse, mental health provider, or registered nutritionist/dietician. Therefore, using and reading this guide does not establish any form of a physician-patient relationship.

Always consult with a physician or another qualified health provider with any issues or questions you might have regarding any sort of medical condition. Do not ever disregard any qualified professional medical advice or delay seeking that advice because of anything you have read in this guide. The information in this guide is not intended to be any sort of medical advice and should not be used in lieu of any medical advice by a licensed and qualified medical professional.

The information in this guide has been compiled from a variety of known sources. However, the author cannot attest to or guarantee the accuracy of each source and thus should not be held liable for any errors or omissions.

You acknowledge that the publisher of this guide will not be held liable for any loss or damage of any kind incurred as a result of this guide or the reliance on any information provided within this guide. You acknowledge and agree that you assume all risk and responsibility for any action you undertake in response to the information in this guide.

Using this guide does not guarantee any particular result (e.g., weight loss or a cure). By reading this guide, you acknowledge that there are no guarantees to any specific outcome or results you can expect.

All product names, diet plans, or names used in this guide are for identification purposes only and are the property of their respective owners. The use of these names does not imply endorsement. All other trademarks cited herein are the property of their respective owners.

Where applicable, this guide is not intended to be a substitute for the original work of this diet plan and is, at most, a supplement to the original work for this diet plan and never a direct substitute. This guide is a personal expression of the facts of that diet plan.

Where applicable, persons shown in the cover images are stock photography models and the publisher has obtained the rights to use the images through license agreements with third-party stock image companies.

# Table of Contents

**Introduction**   7
**Understanding Microdosing**   9
   What Is Microdosing and How Does It Work?   9
   Potential Benefits: PTSD Relief, Mood Stabilization, and Cognitive Clarity   11
   Risks, Side Effects, and Who Should Avoid It   13
   How Microdosing Differs from Full Psychedelic Trips   16
**Setting Up Your Grow Space**   20
   Choosing the Right Mushroom Species (Psilocybe Cubensis & Others)   20
   Essential Equipment and Materials   22
   Preparing a Clean and Sterile Environment   24
   Legal and Safety Considerations   26
**The Beginner's 3-Week Step-by-Step Microdosing & Growing Guide**   28
   Week 1: Preparation & Cultivation Basics   28
   Week 2: Monitoring Growth & Starting Microdosing   34
   Week 3: Harvesting, Dosing, and Long-Term Benefits   40
**Optimizing Microdosing for Mental Health**   57
   Best Practices for PTSD, Depression, and Anxiety   57
   Combining Microdosing with Therapy & Meditation   59
   Nutrition and Lifestyle Adjustments to Maximize Benefits   61
**Troubleshooting and Safety Precautions**   64
   Common Mistakes in Growing and Microdosing   64
   How to Identify and Handle Contaminated Batches   66
   What to Do If You Have a Negative Experience   68
**Legal, Ethical, and Future Perspectives**   71
   The Evolving Legal Landscape of Psilocybin   71
   Ethical Considerations in Psychedelic Use   73
   Future Research and Medical Applications   75

**Resources and Further Reading**    77
    Recommended Books and Scientific Studies    77
    Online Communities and Support Networks    79
    Next Steps in Your Psychedelic Journey    81
**Conclusion**    84
**FAQs**    86
**References and Helpful Links**    89

# Introduction

Microdosing has become a topic of growing interest in recent years. People are exploring it as a way to enhance creativity, improve focus, and boost overall well-being—without the intense effects associated with a full dose of certain substances. Essentially, microdosing involves taking very small amounts of substances like magic mushrooms or LSD. The goal isn't to "trip" but to experience subtle shifts in mood or performance that add value to everyday life.

The appeal lies in its potential to bring balance and clarity, especially for those who feel bogged down by stress or burnout. Some say it sharpens their mental edge or helps them reconnect with a sense of joy. Others are curious about its possible benefits for mental health, such as battling anxiety or depression. While scientific research is catching up, many anecdotal reports keep fueling excitement about what microdosing may offer.

However, it's important to approach microdosing responsibly. Without the right knowledge and guidance, it can lead to unintended consequences.

In this guide, we will talk about the following:

- Understanding Microdosing
- Setting Up Your Grow Space
- The Beginner's 3-Week Step-by-Step Microdosing & Growing Guide
- Optimizing Microdosing for Mental Health
- Troubleshooting and Safety Precautions
- Legal, Ethical, and Future Perspectives
- Resources and Further Reading

Whether someone is new to the concept or simply looking for more clarity, this guide aims to provide practical, easy-to-understand insights. By the end of it, readers can walk away with a thorough understanding of how microdosing works and whether it's the right choice for them.

# Understanding Microdosing

Microdosing has captured the curiosity of many as a potential way to enhance mental clarity, emotional balance, and overall well-being. But what exactly is it, how does it work, and is it right for everyone? This chapter breaks it all down into easy-to-digest sections to help readers gain a solid understanding of the practice.

## What Is Microdosing and How Does It Work?

Microdosing involves taking a very small, sub-perceptual dose of a psychedelic substance, like psilocybin mushrooms or LSD, on a structured schedule. A "sub-perceptual" dose means it's small enough that you don't experience a full psychedelic trip or hallucinations. You stay entirely functional and can continue with daily activities.

The theory behind microdosing is that these small doses can subtly interact with brain chemistry to create benefits such as improved mood, better concentration, and reduced symptoms of anxiety or depression—without overwhelming your senses.

**The Science Behind Microdosing**

Psychedelics like psilocybin mushrooms work primarily by interacting with serotonin receptors in the brain, particularly the 5-HT2A receptor. Serotonin is a neurotransmitter responsible for mood regulation, among other things.

When taken in microdoses, psilocybin may gently stimulate these receptors, potentially helping to form new neural connections or pathways. Some researchers and enthusiasts believe that this enhances creativity, emotional resilience, and mental flexibility—allowing people to approach daily challenges with a fresh perspective.

It's important to note that the scientific community is still in the early stages of studying microdosing. While anecdotal reports suggest promising effects, more rigorous research is needed to confirm these findings.

**How Does It Work Day-to-Day?**

Microdosing isn't a one-time thing; it typically involves following a specific schedule. For example, some people use the "three days on, two days off" protocol, while others prefer the "one day on, two days off" method.

The idea is to avoid building tolerance to the substance while allowing the effects to subtly unfold over time. Most users describe feeling "lighter" or "sharper" on the days they microdose, but it's crucial to listen to your body—you shouldn't feel drastically different. If you do, your dose may be too high!

## Potential Benefits: PTSD Relief, Mood Stabilization, and Cognitive Clarity

Microdosing has gained recognition for its potential to support mental well-being and personal development. Its reported benefits range from easing symptoms of PTSD and anxiety to improving mood and enhancing cognitive function. Here's a closer look at these potential effects:

1. **PTSD and Anxiety Relief**

   For individuals struggling with PTSD or anxiety, microdosing may provide relief by helping to regulate emotions and reduce the intensity of stress responses. It is suggested that psilocybin's interaction with serotonin receptors can promote a sense of calm and emotional balance.

Microdosing allows for these benefits without the intensity or overwhelming nature of a full psychedelic experience, making it a more approachable option for people seeking better emotional management.

2. **Mood Stabilization**

   Many people turn to microdosing as a natural way to lift their mood and counteract feelings of depression or negative thought patterns. It appears to help by gently shifting emotional perspectives, improving the ability to enjoy daily life, and fostering a more positive mental outlook. For those caught in cycles of low energy or gloom, microdosing may offer a subtle yet meaningful improvement in day-to-day mood stability.

### 3. Enhanced Cognitive Clarity and Creativity

Another key appeal of microdosing is its potential to enhance cognitive function. Users often report feeling more focused and mentally clear, which can make tasks feel more manageable and enjoyable.

There's also growing interest in how microdosing might spark creativity, helping individuals think outside the box and identify novel solutions. While major strides in productivity aren't guaranteed, this subtle boost in mental sharpness and clarity could provide a useful edge in everyday life.

Beyond specific benefits like easing PTSD or improving mood, microdosing has broader potential for building emotional and mental resilience. This means you may find it easier to handle stress or face challenges with a greater sense of calm and adaptability. With time, microdosing could contribute to a more balanced and empowered state of mind.

While the benefits described here are exciting, they can vary from person to person. Approach microdosing with curiosity and care, being mindful of how it impacts your own mental state over time.

# Risks, Side Effects, and Who Should Avoid It

While microdosing has gained popularity for its potential benefits, it is not without its risks and side effects. To make informed decisions, it's essential to understand these possible pitfalls and recognize if microdosing is right—or not right—for you.

**Potential Risks and Side Effects**

Microdosing is often described as a subtle and manageable experience, but even small doses of psychedelics can come with disadvantages. Here are some common risks and side effects to keep in mind:

- *Tolerance Development:* Taking psilocybin or other psychedelics frequently can cause your body to build tolerance. As tolerance increases, the effects of microdosing may weaken, pushing you to take more. Following proper schedules with built-in rest days is essential to avoid this issue.
- *Physical Discomfort:* Some people experience mild physical side effects, such as nausea, headaches, or stomach upset. These symptoms are typically short-lived but can be unpleasant enough to disrupt your routine.
- *Worsened Anxiety or Mood Instability:* Not everyone reacts positively to psychedelics, even at microdose levels. For some, especially those prone to anxiety or

sensitive to stress, microdosing may intensify negative emotions or create unease.

- ***Complications with Medication:*** Microdosing can interact negatively with certain medications, particularly antidepressants such as SSRIs, or other substances that affect serotonin levels. Combining these could lead to adverse effects or reduce the effectiveness of either the medication or the microdose.
- ***Unpredictable Effects:*** Every individual's neurochemistry is unique, meaning that outcomes can vary widely. While many people report positive experiences, some might not notice any benefits or could experience unexpected side effects.

It's crucial to acknowledge the legal status of psilocybin in your area. Although research into its medical use is growing, psychedelics remain illegal in many jurisdictions. Be aware of the potential legal risks and penalties associated with possession or use. Additionally, sourcing psilocybin responsibly is essential for ensuring safety and quality.

**Who Should Avoid Microdosing?**

Microdosing is not suitable for everyone, and some groups should approach it with extra caution—or avoid it entirely:

- ***Individuals with a History of Psychosis or Schizophrenia:*** Psychedelics can exacerbate

symptoms of psychotic disorders and destabilize those with a predisposition to conditions like schizophrenia. If you have a personal or family history of these disorders, microdosing is strongly discouraged.
- ***Pregnant or Breastfeeding Individuals:*** There is little to no research on the effects of microdosing during pregnancy or breastfeeding. To avoid potential risks, it's best to steer clear of psychedelics during these significant life stages.
- ***Those Taking Certain Medications:*** People taking antidepressants, mood stabilizers, or anti-anxiety medications should consult a healthcare professional before considering microdosing. The interaction between psilocybin and these drugs could lead to unwanted side effects or reduced effectiveness of either treatment.
- ***People in Unstable Mental or Emotional States:*** If you are currently going through a period of extreme stress, trauma, or emotional instability, microdosing might not be the best choice. While it may appeal as a potential solution, addressing underlying issues with the help of a therapist or mental health professional is a safer and more reliable first step.
- ***Minors:*** Microdosing is intended for informed and responsible adults. Psychedelics can affect developing brains in ways that are not fully understood, making it unsuitable for anyone under the age of 18.

Before you begin, take time to thoroughly research and, if possible, consult a healthcare professional, particularly if you have pre-existing medical concerns. Start with the smallest possible dose and monitor your mental and physical reactions closely. Respect the substance, follow schedules responsibly, and prioritize your overall safety and well-being.

Microdosing can be a powerful tool for some, but it is not a guaranteed fix or universally safe practice. By understanding the risks and knowing when to avoid it, you can make sound decisions and explore this practice responsibly.

## How Microdosing Differs from Full Psychedelic Trips

Microdosing and full psychedelic trips are two entirely different approaches to using substances like psilocybin mushrooms, both in terms of experience and purpose. While they stem from the same source, their effects and usages are worlds apart. If you're new to microdosing, it's important to understand these differences to set proper expectations and goals.

**Dosage**

The most obvious difference lies in the amount of the substance consumed. **Microdosing** involves taking a very small, **"sub-perceptual"** dose of psilocybin or another psychedelic substance. These doses typically range from 0.1

to 0.3 grams of dried mushrooms. Such a tiny dose is not meant to create any noticeable changes in perception or intense effects.

Full **psychedelic trips**, on the other hand, involve significantly **larger doses**—commonly starting at 2 grams or more. At these levels, the substance produces powerful, often overwhelming effects that can completely alter your consciousness. The higher the dose, the more profound and immersive the experience becomes.

**Effects**

Microdosing is meant to **produce subtle yet consistent benefits** like improved mood, better focus, and increased emotional resilience. Importantly, there are no hallucinations, no sense of detachment from reality, and no dramatic shifts in perception. The effects are so faint that you may hardly notice anything beyond feeling a little lighter, sharper, or calmer.

A full trip, however, can be deeply intense and transformative. During a **psychedelic experience**, your **senses heighten**, your **perception of time and space shifts**, and your **thoughts may take on a dream-like quality**. Many people experience vivid visuals, such as patterns or colors, as well as strong emotional releases or even a feeling of merging with the universe. Trips can last anywhere from 4-8 hours, often leaving individuals physically and mentally drained afterward.

**Purpose**

The goals behind microdosing and tripping are also quite different. **Microdosing** is often used as a **tool for personal growth, mental clarity, and subtle emotional enhancement**. It is more of a daily or weekly practice aimed at steady improvements over time, blending seamlessly with your everyday life.

Full **psychedelic trips** are typically sought for **profound introspection, spiritual exploration, or emotional breakthroughs**. They are not suited for everyday routines because of their overpowering nature. Instead, they often require intention-setting, preparation, and a safe, controlled environment. The insights they offer can be life-changing, but they demand deep reflection and integration afterward.

**Approachability**

**Microdosing** is seen as a more **approachable option**, particularly for beginners. Due to its mild effects, you can experiment cautiously and evaluate its potential benefits without fear of losing control. It allows you to engage with psychedelics in a functional, manageable way.

Conversely, **full trips** require a much **higher level of preparation, mental readiness, and a supportive environment**. They are not for everyone, as they can sometimes evoke fear, confusion, or difficult emotions. For those unprepared or in unstable mental health states, the risk of negative experiences is significant.

To put it simply, microdosing is like dipping your toes into the water, while a full psychedelic trip is like plunging into the deep end. One is about subtle improvements that integrate into daily life, while the other is about powerful shifts that can transform your perspective altogether. Understanding these distinctions can help you choose the path that aligns best with your needs, goals, and comfort level.

# Setting Up Your Grow Space

Creating the perfect grow space is an essential step in cultivating psilocybin mushrooms successfully. With careful planning, the right tools, and a clean environment, you can create ideal conditions for your mushrooms to thrive. This chapter will guide you through everything you need to know, from choosing the right species to ensuring safety and legality.

## Choosing the Right Mushroom Species (Psilocybe Cubensis & Others)

When it comes to starting your growing journey, selecting the right mushroom species is a critical first decision. Not all mushrooms are equal, and some are better suited for beginners due to their resilience and ease of cultivation.

### Psilocybe Cubensis

Psilocybe cubensis is, by far, the most popular species for beginners. These mushrooms are known for their adaptability and ability to grow in a wide range of settings. They thrive on substrates like brown rice flour, manure, or coconut coir and tolerate minor mistakes better than many other species. They're often referred to as the "beginner's psychedelic mushroom" for a reason—they're forgiving and reliable, making them an excellent starting point.

Cubensis also comes in many strains, like Golden Teacher, B+, and Ecuadorian. These strains differ slightly in appearance, potency, and growth patterns, but as a beginner, you can select any strain that appeals to you.

**Other Species**

While Psilocybe cubensis is the go-to choice, there are other species worth considering if you're feeling adventurous or have specific goals:

- ***Psilocybe cyanescens (aka Wavy Caps):*** Known for their potency, these mushrooms are more challenging to grow because they require colder temperatures and a specific outdoor setup.
- ***Psilocybe tampanensis (aka Magic Truffles):*** This species produces sclerotia, nutrient-rich underground *structures that are easier to cultivate indoors but less visually striking.*
- ***Psilocybe azurescens:*** One of the most potent psilocybin-containing species but difficult to grow indoors. They thrive in outdoor environments and require careful preparation.

Ultimately, Psilocybe cubensis is highly recommended for your first attempt, but understanding the diversity of options can guide your choices as you gain experience.

## Essential Equipment and Materials

Cultivating psilocybin mushrooms requires a few key items to create an ideal growing environment. Think of this as your equipment checklist—having these items on hand will set you up for success.

1. **Substrate Materials**

   The substrate is the material where your mushrooms will grow. For beginners, brown rice flour (BRF) is a popular choice, often used alongside vermiculite and water. Other substrates include coconut coir, horse manure, or even enriched sawdust, depending on the species.

2. **Jars or Containers**

   You'll need containers to hold your substrate and spores for the initial colonization process. Wide-mouth mason jars are commonly used, as they allow good airflow and make it easy to remove colonized substrate later.

3. **Spore Syringes or Liquid Cultures**

   These contain the mushroom spores that will inoculate your substrate. Purchase from a trusted supplier to ensure high-quality, uncontaminated spores or cultures.

4. **Sterilization Tools**

   Cleanliness is crucial (more on this later). Essential sterilization equipment includes:

   - A pressure cooker for sterilizing substrate materials and jars. (If you don't have one, a large pot can sometimes work in a pinch, though it's less effective.)
   - 70% isopropyl alcohol for wiping down surfaces and equipment.
   - A flame source, such as a lighter or alcohol lamp, for sterilizing needles.

5. **Growing Chambers**

   After the substrate is colonized, you'll need a fruiting chamber to create the humid environment mushrooms need to grow. Many people use a clear plastic storage bin modified with ventilation holes. The chamber can also contain perlite or a humidifier to maintain ideal moisture levels.

6. **Thermometer and Hygrometer**

   Temperature and humidity are critical for successful cultivation. A basic thermometer and hygrometer will help you monitor and control these variables.

7. **Workstation Setup**

   This is where you'll do all your work, like preparing jars and inoculating spores. It should be a clean, well-lit, and easily sterilizable surface.

Having the proper tools and materials from the start sets the stage for a smooth growing process.

## Preparing a Clean and Sterile Environment

Mushrooms, while resilient, are surprisingly vulnerable to contamination. Mold, bacteria, and other competitors can quickly take over if hygiene standards aren't rigorously maintained. A clean and sterile environment is your best defense.

1. **Sterilizing Your Equipment**

   Before starting any part of the process, sterilize everything. Your jars or containers, growing chamber, tools, and even the substrate need to be cleaned thoroughly. Use isopropyl alcohol to wipe down surfaces and sterilize needles and lids. A pressure cooker can steam-sterilize jars and substrate materials, killing off contaminants before adding your spores.

2. **Personal Hygiene**

Contamination often comes from the grower themselves. When working in your grow space, make sure to:

- Wash your hands thoroughly with soap and water.
- Wear gloves and sterilize them with alcohol regularly.
- Use a face mask to avoid breathing bacteria or mold spores onto your materials.

3. **The Role of Airflow**

Airborne contaminants are a common threat. To minimize this risk, work in an area with limited airflow. You might consider building a makeshift still-air box—a sealed plastic container with arm holes—that allows you to work in a controlled, contamination-free environment.

4. **Environmental Conditions**

The ideal temperature range for Psilocybe cubensis is between 75-77°F (24-25°C). More advanced species may have specific temperature needs, so always research beforehand. Room humidity should also be monitored during fruiting, as mushrooms grow best in environments with 85-95% humidity. Mist your chamber or use a humidifier to maintain these levels.

5. **Avoiding Cross-Contamination**

    If you're growing multiple strains or species, separate them and work on one project at a time. Label each container and be cautious when handling different sets of spores or materials to reduce the risk of cross-contamination.

# Legal and Safety Considerations

Before you even begin setting up your grow space, consider the legal and safety implications. Psilocybin mushrooms remain illegal in many areas, so growing them can carry serious legal risks.

1. *Understanding Local Laws:* Psilocybin laws can vary widely depending on your location. While some countries or cities have decriminalized possession, growing fungi may still be considered a criminal offense. Always research and understand the relevant laws in your area to avoid unintentionally breaking them.
2. *Discreet Cultivation:* If growing psilocybin mushrooms is not permitted where you live, discretion is key. Keep your grow operation private—avoid sharing details with people unnecessarily, and ensure

the grow area is out of sight from visitors or housemates.
3. ***Personal Safety:*** Never consume mushrooms without verifying their species and dosage. Make sure all mushrooms harvested are correctly identified—psilocybin mushrooms have distinct features, but accidental poisoning from other fungi is a real danger. When in doubt, consult a mycology expert or rely on tested spore sources.
4. ***Responsible Usage:*** Remember that psilocybin is a powerful substance. Always approach it with respect, moderation, and an informed mindset. Growing should be undertaken not just for personal benefit but with a sense of responsibility for your safety and mental well-being.

By following these guidelines, you'll be ready to set up a productive and efficient grow space. With the right preparation and a commitment to cleanliness and safety, you're well on your way to cultivating a successful harvest in the chapters ahead.

# The Beginner's 3-Week Step-by-Step Microdosing & Growing Guide

Starting your microdosing and mushroom cultivation adventure can feel like a big step, but breaking it down into manageable weeks simplifies the process. This chapter focuses on Week 1, guiding you through preparation and the basics of cultivation. By following this structure, you'll build a strong foundation for successful growing and mindful microdosing.

## Week 1: Preparation & Cultivation Basics

This week is all about laying the groundwork. From setting personal goals to setting up your grow space, these first steps are crucial for a rewarding experience.

### Day 1–2: Understanding Your Goals

Before you get your hands dirty, take some time to reflect on why you're embarking on this path. Setting clear intentions helps guide both your microdosing experience and growing process.

## Identifying Your Mental Health Goals

Think about what you hope to achieve with microdosing. Are you looking to reduce anxiety? Improve focus? Cultivating a balanced, grounded mindset? Whatever the reason, write down your motivations. This will serve as a reference point throughout your microdosing practice.

Ask yourself questions like:

- What area of my life would I like to improve?
- How do I hope to feel in a month? Six months?
- Am I addressing personal growth, professional performance, or emotional well-being?

Being specific gives you something measurable to track over time.

## Tracking Baseline Mood and Symptoms

To monitor the benefits of microdosing, start by gauging your current state. Spend these two days journaling about your mood, focus, sleep quality, energy, and any mental health symptoms you're experiencing. Use a simple rating system (such as 1–10) to quantify things like stress, anxiety, or concentration.

Optional tools:

- Use a notebook or a digital app to record this information daily.
- Reflect not just on the negatives but also on moments you feel content or productive.

These baseline observations will give you valuable context as you begin microdosing later.

**Day 3–5: Setting Up Your Grow Environment**

With clear goals in mind, it's time to prepare for cultivation. Creating the right environment and gathering essential supplies ensures your project gets off to a strong start.

**Preparing Spores or Spore Syringes**

Before you begin growing, you'll need spores to start the process. If using spore syringes:

1. Purchase from a trusted supplier to ensure quality and avoid contamination risks.
2. Store the syringes in a cool, dark place like the refrigerator until you're ready to use them.

If you're working with spore prints (instead of syringes), you'll first need to create a sterile liquid culture. This involves mixing spores into sterilized water and transferring them to a syringe under clean conditions.

**Setting Up a Sterile Grow Chamber**

Creating a sterile space is one of the most important steps in mushroom cultivation. Follow these instructions:

1. Select a container for your grow chamber, such as a clear plastic storage bin with ventilation holes.
2. Wipe it down thoroughly with 70% isopropyl alcohol to eliminate contaminants.
3. Consider lining the bottom with perlite, which helps maintain high humidity levels during fruiting.
4. Place the chamber in a clean, temperature-stable room away from direct sunlight or heavy foot traffic.

Always keep tools like gloves, alcohol wipes, and a flameless lighter (for sterilizing needles) nearby.

**Choosing the Right Substrate**

The substrate is home to your growing mushrooms. For beginners, brown rice flour (BRF) combined with vermiculite and water is a highly reliable option. Here's how to prepare it:

1. Mix the substrate in a bowl using the recommended ratio for your jars (usually 2 parts vermiculite, 1 part BRF, and just enough water to dampen it without puddles forming).
2. Fill clean mason jars loosely with this mixture and top it with a layer of dry vermiculite as a barrier against contaminants.

**Proper Temperature and Humidity Control**

Mushrooms thrive under precise conditions. Psilocybe cubensis, for example, prefers these settings:

- Temperature during colonization: 75–80°F (24–27°C). A stable room temperature usually works, but a small heater might help if your space is cold.
- Humidity during fruiting (later in the process): 85–95%. You won't need this right away, but plan to mist your chamber or use a humidifier when the time comes.

A thermometer and hygrometer are critical for monitoring these variables.

### Day 6–7: Beginning the Growth Process

Now that your environment and materials are ready, it's time to begin the growth process by inoculating your substrate.

### Inoculating the Substrate with Spores

This step introduces spores to the prepared substrate and kickstarts the colonization process:

1. Sterilize your jars and substrate using a pressure cooker. Allow them to cool completely before handling.
2. Flame-sterilize your spore syringe needle until it glows red. Allow the needle to cool briefly.
3. Insert the syringe needle into the jar (through pre-drilled holes in the lid, if applicable). Gently inject

spore solution into 3–4 different spots, distributing it evenly for better colonization.
4. Seal the jar, ensuring the vermiculite layer remains undisturbed. Do not over-tighten the lid or airflow may be restricted.

## **Placing in Incubation with Controlled Conditions**

After inoculation, store the jars in a warm, stable environment to encourage colonization. Tips for success:

- Place your jars in a dark location, such as an enclosed cupboard.
- Maintain temperatures of 75–80°F (24–27°C) to speed up colonization.
- Avoid moving the jars around unnecessarily as this can disturb growth.

Within a few days to a week, you should notice white, fluffy mycelium beginning to form. This network will eventually colonize the entire substrate.

## **Understanding Contamination Risks and How to Prevent Them**

Contamination is the biggest threat to success. Here's how to avoid it:

- Use gloves and a mask when handling materials to minimize bacteria transfer.

- Work in a clean area, wiping surfaces and tools with alcohol before use.
- Inspect your jars daily for signs of mold (red, green, or black spots). If contamination appears, discard the jar immediately to prevent spreading.

By the end of Week 1, your jars will be in the early stage of colonization. You've taken the first major step on your growing and microdosing journey—great progress! Week 2 will build on this foundation, moving closer to a fully developed grow. Keep your excitement high but your patience steady—the best is yet to come!

## Week 2: Monitoring Growth & Starting Microdosing

At this point, your mushroom cultivation should be showing progress, and you're ready to take the first steps into microdosing. This week will involve monitoring colonization for signs of health and contamination, preparing for the first harvest, and beginning your microdosing practice. Here's how to tackle each day with confidence and care.

### Day 8–9: Checking on Mushroom Colonization

Your jars have been incubating for about a week, and it's time to inspect their progress. Monitoring colonization is crucial to ensure healthy growth and identify any issues early.

**Recognizing Healthy vs. Contaminated Growth**

Healthy colonization is marked by a fluffy, white layer of mycelium spreading evenly throughout the substrate. It should look like a web-like network gradually overtaking the surface. Here's what to look for:

- *Healthy signs:* Bright white mycelium with no discoloration or unusual textures.
- *Contamination signs:* Any green, black, red, or yellow spots suggest mold or bacteria. Contaminated jars should be discarded immediately to prevent spreading.

Give each jar a thorough visual inspection daily. If in doubt, compare your jars to photos of healthy versus contaminated colonization (easily found through online mushroom grow communities).

## Adjusting Humidity and Airflow

The colonization stage thrives in a slightly humid and stable environment with limited airflow to reduce contamination risks. Check that:

- The jars are sealed but not overly tight, allowing slight gas exchange through filters or inoculation holes.
- The grow chamber's humidity levels are consistent, and there's no pooling water in the jars.

If conditions feel too dry, you can lightly mist the inside of the grow chamber (not the jars directly) to regulate humidity.

Avoid drastic changes, as mushrooms prefer a steady environment.

**Day 10–11: Preparing for First Harvest**

By now, your mycelium should be nearing full colonization, and pinning—the first signs of mushroom fruiting—may begin soon. This is an exciting stage as your work starts to show visible progress.

**<u>Understanding Pinning (Mushroom Formation)</u>**

Pins are tiny mushroom "buds" that form when the mycelium begins to fruit. These look like small white or brownish bumps on the surface of the substrate. Here's what you need to know:

- Pinning is triggered by increased airflow, lower $CO_2$ levels, and exposure to light, so you'll need to transition the jars to fruiting conditions.
- If you don't see pins yet, don't panic. Some strains take longer than others, but maintaining proper temperature and humidity will encourage pinning.

**<u>Introducing Fresh Air Exchange</u>**

To support healthy fruiting, start introducing fresh air exchange (FAE) into the chamber while maintaining high humidity:

1. Remove the jar lids and, if the mycelium is solid and fully colonized, carefully transfer the colonized substrate into the fruiting chamber.
2. Adjust ventilation in your fruiting chamber by opening vents or fanning it lightly 2–3 times a day. Do this in a clean environment to avoid introducing contaminants.
3. Keep the humidity at 85–95% by misting the chamber walls with clean water. Monitor with a hygrometer to ensure consistency.

Light also plays a role during this stage. Indirect daylight or a 12-hour light/dark cycle with a low-intensity light source typically works well.

## Day 12: Introduction to Microdosing

With your cultivation progressing, it's time to gently introduce yourself to microdosing. Starting this practice allows you to explore its potential benefits while staying mindful and measured.

### **Choosing Your First Microdose Amount**

A typical microdose of psilocybin is about 1/20 to 1/10 of a recreational dose. For beginners, a range of 0.1 to 0.3 grams of dried mushrooms is often recommended. Start on the lower end of the range and adjust as needed in future doses.

To measure your dose:

1. Use a digital scale to weigh the mushrooms precisely. Avoid estimating to ensure safety and consistency.
2. If you're using fresh mushrooms, note that they contain about 90% water compared to dried ones. Adjust the weight accordingly (e.g., 1 gram of dried mushrooms is equivalent to around 10 grams fresh).

## Best Practices: When and How to Take It

Timing and setting are key to a positive microdosing experience:

- ***Best time:*** Many people prefer mornings with breakfast, as this minimizes the chance of affecting sleep and allows you to notice effects throughout the day.
- ***How to take it:*** You can consume the mushrooms as they are, mix them into a smoothie, or brew them into a tea. Choose whatever feels most comfortable.

Start on a day when you have light responsibilities, so you can focus on how you feel without unnecessary pressure.

## Common Effects and What to Expect

Microdosing is subtle and shouldn't feel overwhelming. Common effects may include:

- A mildly elevated mood or sense of lightness
- Increased focus or creativity
- A more relaxed attitude toward daily challenges

You should not experience hallucinations, distortion, or a "high." If you do, your dose may be too high, and you'll want to reduce it next time.

**Day 13–14: Tracking Your Response**

Now that you've taken your first microdose, this part of the week focuses on observing and adjusting. Microdosing is as much about reflection as it is about the substance.

1. **Keeping a Microdosing Journal**

    Documenting your experience helps you understand how microdosing affects you over time. Use your journal to track:

    - The date, time, and dosage of each microdose
    - How you feel before, during, and after taking it
    - Any noticeable changes in mood, productivity, anxiety, or focus

    Consistency is key. Even subtle changes may become clear when you compare journal entries over time.

2. **Noting Changes in Mood, Anxiety, or Focus**

    Pay close attention to shifts in the mental health goals you identified earlier. Questions to guide your reflection:

    - Did you feel more or less productive today?

- How did you respond to stress compared to usual?
- Were there moments of unexpected joy or clarity?

If no changes are apparent yet, don't worry—it can take several days or weeks to notice the cumulative effects.

3. **<u>Adjusting Dosage if Necessary</u>**

Everyone is unique, so it might take a few attempts to find your ideal microdose. If you feel nothing at all, increase your next dose slightly (e.g., from 0.1 g to 0.15 g). If you feel too much, try reducing it. The goal is to find a balance where the benefits feel natural and integrated into daily life.

By the end of Week 2, you'll have made significant progress in both cultivation and microdosing. With colonization progressing and your microdosing practice started, Week 3 will focus on harvest and integrating the practice into your life.

# Week 3: Harvesting, Dosing, and Long-Term Benefits

In this week, we will cover the final steps in the process of cultivating psychedelic mushrooms and incorporating microdosing into your routine.

**Day 15–16: Harvesting Your First Mushrooms**

You've reached one of the most exciting milestones—harvesting your first mushrooms! This stage requires close attention to detail to ensure the mushrooms are collected at their prime and stored properly for future use. Here's how to complete these crucial steps successfully.

**How to Tell When Mushrooms Are Ready for Harvest:**

Timing your harvest is essential for both potency and quality. You'll know your mushrooms are ready when they reach optimal maturity. Here's what to look for:

1. ***Check the Caps:*** The most reliable indicator is the veil—the thin membrane connecting the cap to the stem. Harvest when the veil begins to break, revealing the gills underneath the cap. Waiting too long can result in the cap flattening or even releasing spores, which isn't necessarily bad but may impact taste and appearance.
2. ***Size and Shape:*** Mushrooms are often harvested when the caps are still slightly convex (curved downward), rather than fully flattened. However, size isn't the primary concern, so focus on the veil rather than the height of the mushroom.
3. ***Daily Monitoring:*** Once you see pins growing into full mushrooms, check them at least twice a day. Mushrooms can mature quickly, sometimes overnight,

so keeping an eye on them helps you avoid missing the best harvesting moment.

When in doubt, it's better to harvest slightly early than too late. Early mushrooms still offer full potency and are easier to handle.

**Proper Drying and Storage Methods**

After harvesting, you'll need to dry your mushrooms to preserve their potency and prevent spoilage. Proper storage ensures they remain effective and safe for long-term use. Follow these steps:

1. **Harvesting**
    - Use clean hands or gloves and sterilize any tools (like scissors or knives) with alcohol.
    - Gently twist and pull the mushroom from the substrate. If the stem remains stubbornly attached, use sterilized scissors to cut it as close to the base as possible.
    - Brush off any excess substrate or debris, but avoid washing the mushrooms, as water can cause them to rot.
2. **Drying Mushrooms:** Drying removes moisture, which is essential for long-term storage. Here's the process:
    - *Air Drying (Initial Step):* Place your mushrooms on a clean paper towel or a wire rack in a cool, shaded, and well-ventilated area.

Arrange them in a single layer to ensure airflow. Allow them to air dry for 24–48 hours, or until they become noticeably less pliable.
- ***Using a Dehydrator (Recommended):*** For the best results, use a food dehydrator set to a low temperature (95–105°F or 35–40°C) to dry the mushrooms completely. Avoid higher temperatures, as heat can degrade the psilocybin content.
- ***Cracker Dry Stage:*** Dry your mushrooms until they are "cracker dry"—meaning they snap easily instead of bending. Any remaining moisture can lead to mold during storage, so this step is vital.

3. **<u>Storing Mushrooms:</u>** Once your mushrooms are fully dry, proper storage will protect them from moisture and air exposure:
    - ***Choose an Airtight Container:*** Use a clean, airtight jar or vacuum-sealed bag to store your mushrooms. Adding a food-safe desiccant packet can help absorb any remaining moisture.
    - ***Store in a Cool, Dark Place:*** Keep the container in a closet, cupboard, or any place that is shielded from sunlight and extreme heat. The optimal storage temperature is below 70°F (21°C).

- ***Optional Freezing:*** For long-term storage, you can freeze dried mushrooms. Place them in a vacuum-sealed bag or airtight container, ensuring they are fully dried first. Freezing can help maintain their potency for years.

If you're growing different strains, label each batch with the species, harvesting date, and any other relevant details. This will help you keep track of what works best for your microdosing practice.

By mastering these harvesting, drying, and storage techniques, you'll ensure your mushrooms stay potent and ready for use whenever you need them.

### Day 17–18: Microdosing Schedule Optimization

By Day 17, you've taken a few microdoses and started observing how your mind and body respond. This is the perfect time to fine-tune your routine to maximize benefits. Microdosing isn't "one-size-fits-all," so optimizing your schedule and dosage can help you find what works best for you. Here's how to approach these key steps.

#### *Adjusting Dosage Based on Personal Response*

Everyone processes psilocybin differently due to factors like metabolism, sensitivity, and lifestyle. Use these two days to reflect on your experiences and dial in your ideal dose:

1. **Review Your Journal Entries:**

Look over the notes you've been taking about your mood, focus, sleep, and general feelings after microdosing. Questions to guide this reflection include:

- Did you feel noticeable improvements?
- Were you too stimulated or not stimulated enough?
- Did the effects last throughout the day?

2. **Make Adjustments as Needed:**
    - If you felt little to no change, consider increasing your dose slightly. For example, if you started at 0.1 grams, try 0.15 grams next.
    - If you found the effects too noticeable or distracting, reduce your dose (e.g., from 0.2 grams to 0.15 grams).
3. **Adjust Gradually:** Avoid making big jumps in dosage all at once. Small increments help you hone in on the right amount without risking any undesirable effects.
4. **Recognize Your Sweet Spot:** The right dose enhances your mood, focus, or creativity subtly. It shouldn't interfere with your daily activities or make you feel "off." Once you've discovered this balance, stick with it consistently.

*Common Microdosing Protocols*

Establishing a schedule is just as important as finding the right dose. Most microdosers follow one of several popular protocols that help maintain effectiveness while giving your body time to reset. Two of the most widely-used methods are the **Fadiman Protocol** and the **Stamets Stack**.

Here's how they work:

### *The Fadiman Protocol*

Developed by Dr. James Fadiman, this schedule is simple and easy to follow:

1. Take a microdose on Day 1.
2. Skip the dose on Days 2 and 3 to allow your body to integrate and reset.
3. Repeat this three-day cycle.

**Why it works:** The breaks between doses prevent tolerance build-up, allowing each microdose to remain effective. It's also ideal for beginners since it provides a consistent yet gentle routine.

### *The Stamets Stack*

Paul Stamets, a renowned mycologist, introduced this protocol, combining psilocybin with additional supplements to enhance cognitive benefits. His approach includes:

1. Microdose every day for four days in a row.
2. Take the next three days off before restarting the cycle.
3. Optional enhancement with the "stack": Lion's Mane mushroom extract and niacin (vitamin B3), which are

believed to support neurogenesis (growth of new brain cells).

**Why it works:** This stack aims to harness psilocybin's effects alongside other natural compounds for increased mental clarity and focus. However, beginners should start with only psilocybin before adding supplements to gauge individual responses.

## *Choosing Your Protocol*

Both protocols are effective, but the best choice depends on your goals and routine:

- If you prefer a slower, more reflective approach, try Fadiman's method.
- If you're seeking a concentrated boost, the Stamets Stack may be a good match.

Whenever you switch or adjust protocols, give it at least 1–2 weeks to observe results.

## *Final Tips*

- **Stay Flexible:** If neither method feels right, create a schedule that fits your unique needs. Just ensure you're taking regular breaks between microdosage days.
- **Track Progress:** Continue journaling to refine both your dose and schedule over time. Patterns will emerge, showing what works best for your mind and body.

By the end of Day 18, you should feel more confident about your microdosing practice. With your ideal dose and schedule in place, you'll be on track to fully enjoy the long-term benefits of microdosing in the days ahead!

**Day 19–20: Understanding Long-Term Benefits**

You've explored the basics of microdosing, fine-tuned your dosage, and started to notice some initial effects. Now it's time to look at the bigger picture—how microdosing can affect your brain and mental well-being over time. Understanding these potential benefits can help you stay motivated and develop a sustainable microdosing practice.

*How Microdosing Affects the Brain Over Time*

Microdosing is thought to encourage positive changes in the brain through mechanisms that enhance connectivity and promote adaptation. While more research is needed, here's what scientists and users believe happens with consistent microdosing:

1. **<u>Neuroplasticity Boost:</u>** Psilocybin, the active compound in magic mushrooms, interacts with serotonin receptors in the brain. This interaction is believed to enhance neuroplasticity, which is the brain's ability to form new neural connections. Over time, this can improve learning, creativity, and adaptability.

2. **Strengthened Brain Connectivity:** Studies suggest that psilocybin increases communication between different areas of the brain, shifting away from rigid patterns of thinking. This can lead to new perspectives, more flexible problem-solving skills, and reduced mental "stuckness," especially for individuals experiencing depression or anxiety.
3. **Improved Emotional Regulation:** By modulating the brain's default mode network (DMN)—the area responsible for self-reflection and rumination—microdosing may reduce overactivity in the DMN, a hallmark in conditions like anxiety and obsessive thinking. Over time, this can promote a calmer, more centered state of mind.

While these effects won't create instant, dramatic changes, the subtle shifts from consistent microdosing can build up into meaningful improvements in cognitive and emotional functioning.

*Potential Long-Term Mental Health Improvements*

Aside from the brain-level effects, many people report significant, long-lasting benefits to their mental health when microdosing over weeks or months. Here are some of the most common improvements:

1. **Reduction in Anxiety and Depression Symptoms:** Microdosing may help lighten the weight of anxiety

and low mood. Users often describe feeling less overwhelmed by negative thoughts and more equipped to manage day-to-day stressors. Over time, this can reinforce a greater sense of stability and well-being.

2. **Improved Focus and Productivity:** Many individuals find that microdosing increases their ability to stay focused and engaged in tasks. Whether you're working on a creative project or managing everyday responsibilities, this improved concentration can lead to greater satisfaction and a sense of accomplishment over the long term.

3. **Enhanced Interpersonal Relationships:** By helping to ease emotional reactivity and encourage empathy, microdosing can lead to easier, more meaningful social interactions. You may find it simpler to communicate, connect, and cultivate healthier dynamics with loved ones and colleagues alike.

4. **Resilience Against Negative Thought Patterns:** Over time, the shifts in perspective brought about by microdosing may help break cycles of negative rumination. This can result in a more optimistic outlook and an improved ability to face challenges with a problem-solving mindset.

In the long run, microdosing may offer meaningful mental health benefits, from reduced anxiety to improved focus and relationships. While individual experiences vary, many users report feeling more balanced, resilient, and empowered in their daily lives.

## *Building Long-Term Benefits into Your Practice*

To maximize the potential long-term benefits of microdosing, it's important to approach the practice mindfully and intentionally. Here are some steps to ensure sustainable progress:

1. **Keep Reflecting on Goals:** The goals you set at the beginning of this guide—whether they relate to mental health, creativity, or productivity—should remain your compass. Regularly review your progress to make sure your practice aligns with these intentions.
2. **Balance Microdosing with Self-Care:** Microdosing is just one tool in a larger framework of well-being. Pair your practice with other healthy habits like exercise, meditation, and a balanced diet to support long-term mental health.
3. **Reassess Regularly:** Take time every few months to evaluate your dosage and schedule. You may find that you need to tweak your approach as your needs and goals evolve.

By Day 20, you'll have a deeper understanding of how microdosing can impact both your brain and your quality of life over time. As you move forward, remember that consistency and mindfulness are your best allies in making lasting, positive changes. The benefits will continue to unfold as long as you remain patient and open to the process.

## Day 21: Reflecting & Planning Next Steps

Day 21 is all about reflecting on your progress so far and deciding where to go next. Taking this time to review your journey can help you make informed, intentional choices as you continue exploring the advantages of microdosing—or perhaps even other therapeutic options.

### *Evaluating Your Progress*

Reflection is key to understanding how much you've gained from this process. Set aside some time to review your microdosing experience and think critically about what's worked for you and what hasn't. Here's how to assess your progress step-by-step:

1. **Review Your Goals and Journal Entries:** Look back at the goals you set on Day 1 and your notes from each microdosing session. Ask yourself:
    - Have you noticed improvements in areas like mood, focus, creativity, or anxiety?
    - Have any unexpected patterns or benefits emerged?
    - Were there any challenges, and if so, were you able to address them?
2. **Recognize Positive Changes:** Even small shifts are worth celebrating! Perhaps you feel more calm and

composed in stressful situations or more connected to creative thinking. These changes often build incrementally, so acknowledging them can motivate you to keep going.

3. **Consider What You'd Like to Improve Further:** If certain goals remain unmet, think about why this might be. For example, is your dosage optimal? Would a different microdosing schedule better suit your needs? Identifying areas for refinement gives you a roadmap for continued growth.

## *Deciding Whether to Continue Microdosing*

At this point, you might be thinking about whether microdosing is something you want to continue long-term. Some people find it very beneficial and make it a regular part of their lives, while others prefer to try different options. Here are some questions to help you decide:

1. **How Have You Felt Overall?**

   If the experience has been overwhelmingly positive and you've noticed meaningful benefits, continuing with microdosing might make sense. On the other hand, if it hasn't met your expectations, it's okay to step back or make adjustments.

2. **Can You Sustain the Practice?**

Ask yourself whether microdosing fits naturally into your lifestyle. If you enjoy the routine and find it manageable, commitment is easier. If not, consider changes to your schedule or dosage—or take a break to re-evaluate later.

3. **Experiment with Pausing:**

    Many people pause microdosing periodically to ensure continued effectiveness and avoid reliance. After completing this guide, you might take a few weeks off, then return to see if the benefits resurface.

Remember, there's no "right" answer—microdosing is a personal and adaptable practice. Your needs and priorities may evolve, and that's perfectly okay.

*Exploring Other Psychedelic Therapies*

If you've enjoyed the subtle effects of microdosing, you might find it worthwhile to learn about other forms of psychedelic therapy. While microdosing provides gentle, daily benefits, other therapies may offer deeper, more impactful experiences for emotional healing or personal growth. Here are some options to research:

1. **Macrodosing/Full Psychedelic Journeys:** A macrodose is a larger dose of psychedelics intended to induce a full-blown psychedelic experience. When done in a safe, supportive environment, these sessions

can provide profound insights and emotional breakthroughs. However, they require careful preparation and guidance.

2. **Guided Psychedelic Therapy:** Programs with trained therapists offer a controlled setting for exploring higher doses of psychedelics like psilocybin or MDMA. These therapies are becoming more widely accepted for treating mental health challenges such as PTSD, depression, and anxiety.

3. **Other Compounds:** Beyond psilocybin, substances like LSD, ketamine, and ayahuasca have shown promise in therapeutic applications. Each option has its risks and benefits, so further research and consultation with professionals are critical.

4. **Nature-Based Healing Practices:** If you feel a connection to the natural origin of psilocybin, you might be intrigued by other plant-based therapies, such as peyote or San Pedro cactus ceremonies. These practices often come with cultural traditions and rituals that add depth to the experience.

*Planning Your Next Steps*

- **Commit to Learning More:** Whether continuing microdosing or exploring other options, make time to educate yourself further. Reliable books, studies, or courses can guide your next steps.

- **Choose a Path That Feels Right:** Follow your intuition about what fits best with your goals, lifestyle, and level of comfort.
- **Connect with a Community:** If possible, seek out supportive groups or knowledgeable individuals to share experiences and ideas.

Reflecting on your journey with microdosing is an important step in understanding its impact and deciding your next steps. Whether you continue microdosing, explore other therapeutic options, or take a pause, the key is to follow a path that aligns with your goals and well-being.

# Optimizing Microdosing for Mental Health

Your microdosing practice can go beyond experimentation and curiosity—it has the potential to support your mental health in powerful ways. If you're dealing with conditions like PTSD, depression, or anxiety, or simply want to boost your emotional well-being, this chapter will show you how to fine-tune your approach.

By following best practices, pairing microdosing with other supportive tools, and making thoughtful lifestyle changes, you can unlock its full benefits.

## Best Practices for PTSD, Depression, and Anxiety

Microdosing is gaining attention for its ability to gently support mental health, including challenging conditions like PTSD, depression, and anxiety. While research is ongoing, many people have found relief through consistent, mindful use of psilocybin. Below are some tips to help you get the most out of microdosing while addressing these conditions.

1. **Start With Small, Consistent Doses**
   - Microdosing involves sub-perceptual doses, meaning you won't feel high or experience hallucinations. For most beginners, a good starting dose is 0.1g–0.3g of dried psilocybin mushrooms.
   - Take your dose in the morning on your chosen schedule (e.g., every other day or 2-3 times per week) and avoid increasing it unless absolutely necessary. Consistency is key.
2. **Keep Track of Your Experience**
   - Journaling is incredibly helpful for observing patterns and progress. Write down how you feel each day, noting any changes in mood, energy, or anxiety levels.
   - Look for trends over time—are you feeling calmer, more focused, or less stuck in negative thought loops?
3. **Be Patient With Progress**
   - Microdosing often brings gentle, gradual improvements rather than overnight transformations. Shift your focus from "fixing" symptoms to noticing small, positive changes over weeks or months.
   - Allow the practice to support you naturally without pressuring yourself to feel a certain way.

4. **Work With a Professional If Possible**
   - If you're dealing with significant PTSD, depression, or anxiety, consider seeking guidance from a trained psychedelic therapist or mental health professional. They can help you determine whether microdosing is a good fit for your situation and monitor your progress safely.

By combining microdosing with mindfulness and patience, many have found it easier to break free from mental health struggles, gain perspective, and move forward with a lighter mindset.

# Combining Microdosing with Therapy & Meditation

Microdosing on its own is powerful, but when paired with complementary practices like talk therapy or meditation, its impact can be even greater. These approaches work together to help you deepen self-awareness, process emotions, and create lasting mental health improvements.

1. **Using Microdosing to Enhance Therapy**
   - Whether you're seeing a therapist weekly or participating in a specific mental health program, microdosing can help you feel more open, reflective, and emotionally connected during these sessions.

- Share your microdosing practice with your therapist (if they're open to it) so they can guide you through any insights or feelings that arise.
- Many people say microdosing allows them to recognize patterns or emotions they hadn't noticed before, making their sessions more productive.

2. **Pairing Meditation With Microdosing**
   - Microdosing can make it easier to get into a calm, focused state for meditation. This is because psilocybin promotes mindfulness and presence by quieting overactive thoughts.
   - Start with basic mindfulness techniques—sit in a quiet space, focus on your breathing, and observe your thoughts without judgment.
   - Consider guided meditations focused on self-compassion or healing, which work beautifully alongside microdosing. Apps like Calm, Headspace, or Insight Timer are great tools to try.

3. **Explore Body-Centered Practices**
   - Yoga, breathwork, or even a simple nature walk can complement your microdosing routine. The combination of movement and mindfulness boosts relaxation and helps release tension stored in the body.

- Pay attention to how your body feels after these practices and notice whether microdosing enhances your sense of balance and connection.

The goal is to create an environment of self-care where microdosing is one piece of a larger puzzle for well-being. When combined with therapy or meditation, the results can often feel more profound and rooted.

## Nutrition and Lifestyle Adjustments to Maximize Benefits

What you eat, how you move, and the habits you maintain have a significant influence on the benefits you'll experience with microdosing. By supporting your body and mind through healthy choices, you can amplify psilocybin's effects and enjoy more sustained improvements to your mental health.

1. **Prioritize Brain-Boosting Foods**
    - Include foods rich in omega-3 fatty acids, such as salmon, walnuts, and flaxseeds. These promote brain health and support mood regulation.
    - Look for antioxidant-packed fruits and veggies, like berries, spinach, and kale, which reduce inflammation and improve overall well-being.
    - Avoid processed and sugary foods as much as possible, as they can disrupt mental clarity and mood stability.

2. **Stay Hydrated**
    - Drinking enough water may sound simple, but it's essential. Proper hydration helps with focus, energy, and emotional balance—all things microdosing aims to support.
    - Aim for 8–10 glasses of water a day, and cut back on dehydrating drinks like coffee or alcohol.
3. **Create a Regular Sleep Schedule**
    - Quality sleep is the foundation of good mental health. Make sure you're getting 7–9 hours of rest each night, and try to maintain a consistent bedtime.
    - Consider using your microdosing routine to help balance mornings and establish a calm, intentional start to your day.
4. **Move Your Body Daily**
    - Physical activity naturally boosts serotonin and endorphins, helping you feel better emotionally and physically. Even a 15-minute walk or light stretching can make a difference.
    - Try pairing active moments with your microdosing schedule to create a mental and physical uplift on dosing days.

5. **Limit Toxic Stress**
    - Take note of the things that drain your energy and mood, such as overworking, negative relationships, or constant social media scrolling.
    - Replace these stressors with uplifting activities, like reading, connecting with loved ones, or taking time for hobbies.
6. **Build a Supportive Routine**
    - Structure your days to include intentional moments of self-care, reflection, and mindfulness. This not only supports microdosing but also builds emotional resilience over time.

By bringing these healthy habits into your life, you'll create the ideal conditions for microdosing to thrive. Your mind and body will be more receptive to its benefits, and those benefits will feel more lasting and tangible.

Optimizing your microdosing practice is as much about intention and care as it is about the actual dose. By following best practices for mental health, combining microdosing with grounding techniques like therapy or meditation, and supporting yourself with a healthy lifestyle, you can create a holistic approach to healing and growth.

# Troubleshooting and Safety Precautions

Every new skill comes with a learning curve, and growing mushrooms or starting a microdosing routine is no exception. Mistakes can happen, and while they're part of the process, knowing how to troubleshoot issues and keep yourself safe is essential.

This chapter will guide you through common pitfalls, teach you how to spot contaminated mushrooms, and help you manage any negative experiences with microdosing calmly and effectively.

## Common Mistakes in Growing and Microdosing

To get the best results from your microdosing practice, it's important to avoid some easily preventable mistakes.

1. **Growing Mistakes**
    - ***Skipping Sterilization:*** Contamination often starts because of unclean tools or growing

spaces. Always sterilize everything thoroughly before you begin, including jars, substrate, and work surfaces.
- ***Wrong Temperature or Humidity Conditions:*** Mushrooms thrive in specific conditions. Too much moisture or heat can stunt growth or encourage mold. Keep the temperature around 70–75°F (21–24°C) and monitor humidity closely.
- ***Rushing the Process:*** Patience is crucial. Avoid checking your mushrooms too often or tampering with them unnecessarily. Mushrooms grow best when left undisturbed with consistent care.

2. **Microdosing Mistakes**
   - ***Starting Too High:*** A common beginner mistake is taking too much early on, resulting in noticeable effects that may not feel manageable. Stick to a low dose of 0.1g–0.3g and work your way up only if needed.
   - ***Not Following a Schedule:*** Microdosing randomly or too frequently can lead to diminishing returns. Follow a tried-and-true protocol, such as 1 day on and 2 days off, or another structured schedule that allows your body to rest.

- ***Ignoring Set and Setting:*** Even with low doses, your environment and mindset matter. Avoid microdosing when you feel stressed or distracted, and choose a calm, supportive space to get the best results.
- ***Skipping Reflection:*** Without tracking your experience, it's hard to determine what's working. Journal your progress regularly, noting how you feel on both dosing and non-dosing days.

Keep in mind that mistakes are normal, and each misstep brings an opportunity to learn. With time, you'll develop a steady rhythm that works for you.

## How to Identify and Handle Contaminated Batches

Ensuring the mushrooms you've grown are free from contamination is critical for safety and effectiveness. Contaminants can harm your health and compromise the benefits of your microdosing practice, so it's essential to know the warning signs.

1. **Signs of Contamination**
   - ***Unusual Colors:*** Your mushrooms should generally be white, cream, or light brown. Green, black, or bright yellow spots often signal mold or bacterial contamination.

- ***Strange Textures:*** Slimy or overly moist mushrooms are a bad sign. Healthy mushrooms have a firm, dry appearance.
- ***Offputting Smells:*** Fresh mushrooms should have an earthy, neutral smell. If you notice strong, sour, or unpleasant odors, you're likely dealing with contamination.

2. **Handling Contaminated Batches**
   - ***Discard Immediately:*** If you're unsure whether your mushrooms are contaminated, it's better to be safe than sorry. Dispose of the batch carefully to prevent spreading mold or bacteria.
   - ***Do Not Consume or Salvage:*** Even small contaminated sections can be harmful. Avoid cutting away "bad" parts and consuming what's left. Once contamination spreads, the entire batch is unsafe.
   - ***Review Your Growth Setup:*** Check the cleanliness of your materials and growing environment. Sterilize your jars and tools thoroughly before starting a new batch, and be extra mindful of temperature and humidity going forward.

Regularly inspecting your mushrooms and sticking to meticulous growing practices will help prevent contamination and give you peace of mind.

# What to Do If You Have a Negative Experience

Microdosing is designed to stay below the threshold of noticeable effects, but sometimes things don't go as planned. You might accidentally take too much or find that a particular dose isn't sitting well with you. Negative experiences are usually temporary and manageable with the right approach.

1. **Stay Calm and Grounded**
   - If you feel overwhelmed, remind yourself that it's a temporary reaction and not a life-threatening situation. Most mild to moderate effects wear off within a few hours.
   - Take slow, deep breaths to help calm your nervous system. Focus on the rhythm of your breathing to keep your mind centered.
2. **Shift Your Environment**
   - If possible, change your environment to one that feels safe and soothing. Sit in a quiet room, light a candle, or play calming music.
   - Avoid screens, loud noises, or crowded spaces, which can make discomfort worse.
3. **Reach Out for Support**
   - If you're with a trusted friend or loved one, share how you're feeling. Talking openly can often be a comforting way to ease anxiety or self-doubt.

- If you're alone, consider calling someone you trust for reassurance.

4. **Explore Grounding Activities**
    - Try easy activities that connect you to the present moment, such as feeling the texture of a soft blanket, holding a warm cup of tea, or stepping outside for fresh air.
    - Journaling your emotions can also help you process the experience and put things into perspective.

5. **Lower Your Dose Next Time**

If the reaction was due to taking too high a dose, adjust it downward the next time you microdose. Start small and increase only if needed.

6. **Pause if Necessary**

If microdosing doesn't feel right for you, honor that. You can take a break to reevaluate, experiment with a smaller dose later, or explore other wellness practices.

Knowing how to handle a negative experience helps build confidence and reduces fear around experimenting with microdosing. Ultimately, self-compassion and preparedness are your best tools for navigating challenges.

Troubleshooting is a normal part of growing mushrooms and developing a microdosing routine. By avoiding common pitfalls, keeping an eye out for contamination, and addressing negative experiences calmly, you'll gain more confidence in your practice.

# Legal, Ethical, and Future Perspectives

Psilocybin mushrooms, once shrouded in mystery and stigma, are now gaining mainstream attention as a tool for healing and personal growth. But with this spotlight comes the need to understand the legal, ethical, and scientific perspectives surrounding their use.

This chapter will help you grasp the evolving status of psilocybin, the responsibility that comes with its use, and the exciting discoveries shaping its future.

## The Evolving Legal Landscape of Psilocybin

The legal status of psilocybin is changing rapidly around the world. What was once widely banned is now being reconsidered, with growing calls for legalization and regulation based on its potential health benefits.

1. **Current Legal Status**
    - Many Places Still Prohibit Psilocybin: Psilocybin remains classified as an illegal substance in many countries. Be sure you

understand the laws in your area before growing or using psilocybin mushrooms.
- Decriminalization Efforts: Some cities and regions (e.g., parts of the U.S., like Oregon and Colorado) have decriminalized possession of small amounts of psilocybin, making it a lower priority for law enforcement.
- Medical and Therapeutic Use: Countries like Canada and Australia, as well as certain states in the U.S., are beginning to allow psilocybin for specific therapeutic purposes, like treating clinical depression or PTSD, under controlled conditions.

2. **What This Means for You**
   - Always research the laws governing psilocybin in your area. Even where decriminalization exists, growing or purchasing mushrooms may still carry legal risks.
   - Keep an eye on emerging legislation. The landscape is shifting quickly, and more areas could follow suit in recognizing psilocybin's therapeutic potential.

3. **Advocacy and Education**
   - Grassroots organizations and researchers are working hard to educate the public about the benefits of psilocybin. Consider supporting

these efforts if you're passionate about its responsible use.
- By spreading awareness and reducing stigma, we can pave the way for more informed, compassionate policies in the future.

The future of psilocybin will likely depend not just on changing laws, but on how society approaches its use with care and respect.

## Ethical Considerations in Psychedelic Use

Just because something is available doesn't mean it should be used without thought. One of the most important aspects of working with psychedelics, including psilocybin, is taking ethical responsibility for your choices.

1. **Respecting the Substance**
    - Psychedelics are Not a Shortcut: They are tools for personal growth and healing, not quick fixes. Approach them with curiosity, patience, and humility.
    - Avoid Recreational Misuse: While psilocybin can have joyful effects, using it irresponsibly for thrills or peer pressure can diminish its potential and create harm. Always ensure your intentions are aligned with growth and well-being.

2. **Considering Cultural Roots**
    - Psilocybin mushrooms have been used for centuries in indigenous ceremonies. Acknowledge and respect these traditions, and avoid appropriating practices without understanding their cultural significance.
    - If you choose to work with guides or shamans, support those trained in ethical and culturally sensitive practices.
3. **Your Impact on Others**
    - Be mindful of sharing psychedelics with others, especially people unfamiliar with their effects. Never pressure anyone to participate, and prioritize safety in all group settings.
    - Use discretion when discussing psychedelics publicly. While advocacy is important, oversharing could unintentionally encourage unsafe behaviors or draw unwanted attention.
4. **Environmental Sustainability**
    - Growing psilocybin mushrooms can be eco-friendly, but overharvesting mushrooms from natural locations can deplete wild populations. Stick to cultivating your own supply whenever possible.

Ethical mindfulness ensures that psilocybin use remains safe, sustainable, and rooted in respect for both people and the planet.

# Future Research and Medical Applications

Exciting breakthroughs in psilocybin research are shaping the future of mental health care. Scientists are uncovering its potential to transform how we treat conditions like depression, anxiety, and trauma.

1. **What Research Shows**
   - *Psilocybin-Assisted Therapy:* Early studies show that psilocybin can help with treatment-resistant depression, PTSD, and end-of-life anxiety. When combined with therapy, it creates space for profound emotional healing.
   - *Brain Function and Neuroplasticity:* Psilocybin appears to enhance the brain's ability to rewire itself, promoting flexible thinking and reducing negative thought patterns.
   - *Habit and Addiction Recovery:* Trials suggest psilocybin may support people in quitting smoking, overcoming alcoholism, and breaking other harmful behaviors.
2. **Potential Future Applications**
   - *Wider Access to Treatment:* If clinical trials continue to show success, psilocybin therapy could become a routine option for mental health care. This might include clinics where trained professionals guide therapeutic sessions.

- ***Chronic Pain and Cluster Headaches:*** There's growing interest in how psilocybin might help manage conditions like chronic migraines or other pain-related disorders.
- ***Enhancing Personal Growth:*** Beyond medical use, many believe psilocybin has a role in fostering creativity, connection, and self-awareness—even for those without specific health concerns.

3. **Challenges Ahead**
   - Expanding research requires funding and public support, which can be limited by lingering stigma and legal roadblocks.
   - Safety and regulation will be paramount in ensuring psilocybin therapy is accessible without being exploited or abused.

The road to mainstream acceptance will take time, but the possibilities are promising. By staying informed and advocating for responsible use, you can be part of this exciting shift.

Understanding the legal, ethical, and future perspectives of psilocybin highlights its incredible potential—but also reminds us of the care and responsibility it demands. Laws are evolving, cultural conversations are deepening, and scientific breakthroughs are laying the groundwork for a new era of mental health care.

# Resources and Further Reading

Now that you have a deeper understanding of psilocybin, here are some additional resources to continue learning about this fascinating substance:

## Recommended Books and Scientific Studies

Books and research studies are excellent tools for expanding your understanding of psychedelics. Many authors and scientists have dedicated their work to uncovering the mysteries and benefits of psilocybin, and their insights could be invaluable to your practice.

1. **Books to Get You Started**
   - ***"How to Change Your Mind" by Michael Pollan:*** An engaging read that explores the history, science, and cultural significance of psychedelics, including psilocybin. It's great for beginners who want a well-rounded introduction.
   - ***"The Psychedelic Explorer's Guide" by James Fadiman:*** Written by one of the pioneers of

psychedelic research, this book offers practical advice on safe, intentional use and dives into the concept of microdosing.

- *"Fantastic Fungi" by Paul Stamets:* This visually stunning book highlights the wondrous world of fungi and their benefits and includes accessible information on growing and using mushrooms.
- *"Pollination of Consciousness" by Kalindi Jordan:* A beginner-friendly book that blends personal experiences with insights about the therapeutic and spiritual aspects of psilocybin.

2. **Must-Know Scientific Studies**

While books offer accessible explanations, scientific studies offer the data-backed evidence that continues to legitimize psilocybin as a therapeutic tool.

- *Psilocybin for Depression:* Look into the groundbreaking 2016 Johns Hopkins University study showing the positive effects of psilocybin on depression and anxiety.
- *Neuroplasticity Research:* Explore studies detailing how psilocybin promotes flexible thinking by rewiring neural pathways. A good place to start is research published by Imperial College London's Centre for Psychedelic Research.

- *Microdosing Studies:* Though still emerging, preliminary surveys and trials hint at mood, focus, and creativity benefits. Keep an eye on ongoing research in this space.

3. **Where to Find These Materials**
   - Check your local library to borrow books and support educational access.
   - Browse online retailers like Amazon or independent bookstores for your own copies. Don't forget eBook or audiobook options!
   - For scientific studies, websites like PubMed and ResearchGate are excellent for accessing peer-reviewed papers. Some studies may require a subscription to read in full, but abstracts often provide valuable summaries.

# Online Communities and Support Networks

The psilocybin community is filled with people eager to share their experiences and advice. Joining a supportive group can be incredibly helpful, whether you're troubleshooting, seeking encouragement, or simply wanting to connect with like-minded individuals.

1. **Popular Online Communities**
   - *Reddit:* Subreddits like r/microdosing and r/psilocybin offer a wealth of user experiences, tips, and Q&A threads. Just remember to

approach any advice with caution and do your own research.
- *The Third Wave Community Forum:* A trusted space for microdosers that provides education, user stories, and discussions about the responsible use of psychedelics.
- *Shroomery Forums:* One of the oldest and most active online forums for mushroom cultivation and psychedelic discussions. Great for beginner growers.

2. **Finding Local Meetups or Groups**
    - *Local Psychedelic Societies:* Many cities now have groups that meet to discuss topics like microdosing, mental health, and psychedelic research. Check Meetup.com or Facebook to find one near you.
    - *Workshops or Retreats:* Some organizations offer in-person or virtual workshops to learn more about microdosing or therapeutic approaches to psilocybin use. Be sure they're led by qualified instructors in safe environments.

3. **Support for Challenges or Concerns**
    - *Integration Coaches:* These practitioners specialize in helping individuals process and glean insights from psychedelic experiences, whether micro- or macrodoses.

- ***Mental Health Resources:*** If psilocybin stirs up overwhelming emotions or challenges, seek support from trained therapists, ideally those who incorporate psychedelic-informed approaches.

Connecting with online communities and local support networks can provide valuable guidance and encouragement for those exploring psilocybin responsibly. Remember to approach all advice with discernment and prioritize safety and informed decision-making.

## Next Steps in Your Psychedelic Journey

If you feel ready to go beyond the basics, opportunities to expand your practice await. The key is to remain thoughtful, safe, and intentional at each stage.

1. **Deepen Your Microdosing Practice**
   - ***Advanced Techniques:*** Once you're comfortable with standard microdosing, you might want to explore subtle changes, such as trying a different dosing protocol or pairing microdosing with complementary habits like breathwork or creative exercises.
   - ***Pay It Forward:*** Share what you've learned with others while encouraging mindful, ethical approaches to psychedelics. Your insights might

inspire someone else to begin their own healing or growth.

2. **Experiment with New Approaches**
   - *Varied Psychedelics:* If you're curious, research substances like LSD, mescaline, or DMT. These have unique properties and may offer different perspectives when approached responsibly.
   - *Guided Sessions:* Consider experiencing a full macrodose of psilocybin through a supervised, therapeutic session to explore deeper insights and healing.

3. **Continue Learning**
   - Stay up-to-date with psychedelics' evolving role in mental health, therapy, and wellness. Follow reputable researchers, organizations, and publications to keep growing your understanding.
   - Explore professional training opportunities if you feel called to contribute to this field as a grower, advocate, or informed guide.

4. **Stay Open-Minded**

   Above all, remember that your psychedelic path is unique to you. Every new step brings opportunities to learn, adapt, and contribute.

Your psilocybin and microdosing practice is just one part of a larger, dynamic world of personal growth, discovery, and community. With the resources outlined here, you can deepen your understanding and connect with an inspiring network of people who share your enthusiasm.

# Conclusion

Congratulations on completing this guide! By taking the time to learn about microdosing and growing psilocybin mushrooms, you've embarked on a unique and meaningful journey. This path isn't just about learning new skills—it's about tapping into your potential, improving your well-being, and exploring what it truly means to grow, both literally and figuratively.

Think about how far you've come already. You've learned the basics of microdosing, explored the science behind it, and set clear goals. You've also taken the first steps into cultivation, gaining a deeper understanding of how psilocybin mushrooms grow and thrive. Each effort you've made—whether setting up your grow space or reflecting on your experiences—has brought you closer to unlocking the benefits of this practice. Pat yourself on the back for your commitment and curiosity.

Remember, this is just the beginning. Whether your goal is better focus, emotional balance, or personal growth, what you've learned here equips you to continue moving forward with confidence. Stay patient with yourself and trust the process. Growth, like mushrooms, takes time, effort, and care. Celebrate even the small wins—they're the foundation of long-term change.

Moving forward, stay curious and open-minded. Keep refining your practice, exploring new ideas, and connecting with others on a similar path. There's so much potential waiting for you—both in your personal growth and the ripple effect these mindful practices can have on your life.

Thank you for taking the time to explore this guide. By investing in yourself and making thoughtful, informed choices, you're building a meaningful path toward well-being, creativity, and resilience.

# FAQs

**What is microdosing?**

Microdosing is the practice of taking very small, sub-perceptual doses of substances like psilocybin (from magic mushrooms) or LSD. These doses are too small to cause a "trip" or hallucination but are thought to enhance mood, focus, creativity, and overall well-being in subtle ways.

**What are the potential benefits of microdosing?**

Many people report feeling more focused, creative, and emotionally balanced. Microdosing may help with relieving symptoms of anxiety, depression, or PTSD. Others say it boosts their energy, productivity, or introspection. While research is still growing, anecdotal evidence from users highlights these positive effects.

**Are there any risks to microdosing?**

Yes, microdosing isn't risk-free. Potential side effects include mild nausea, headaches, or feelings of anxiety, especially if the dose is too high. It can also interact with medications like antidepressants. The legal status of psychedelics in many places is another important consideration to keep in mind.

**How do I start microdosing?Ω**

Begin by researching thoroughly and planning your approach. Start with a very small dose (typically 0.1–0.3 grams of dried psilocybin mushrooms) and follow a structured schedule, such as one day on, two days off. Keep a journal to track how you feel and adjust as needed. Ensure your setting is safe and comfortable.

**Will I feel "high" when microdosing?**

No, a true microdose is sub-perceptual, meaning you won't experience intense effects or hallucinations. Most people feel just slightly lighter, more focused, or more positive—if they notice the effects at all.

**Is microdosing legal?**

The legal status of microdosing depends on where you live. Substances like psilocybin and LSD are illegal in many places, though some areas have started to decriminalize possession. Research and be fully aware of the laws in your region.

**Can anyone microdose safely?**

Microdosing isn't suitable for everyone. People with a history of schizophrenia or psychosis, those taking certain medications, or pregnant individuals should avoid it. Always consult a healthcare professional if you have concerns or pre-existing conditions.

# References and Helpful Links

News-Medical. (2019, November 11). What is Psychedelic Microdosing? https://www.news-medical.net/health/What-is-Psychedelic-Microdosing.aspx

Radcliffe, S. (2022, July 21). Microdosing psilocybin mushrooms may improve mental health and mood. Healthline. https://www.healthline.com/health-news/microdosing-psilocybin-mushrooms-may-improve-mental-health-and-mood#:~:text=Microdosing%20psychedelics%20may%20offer%20unique,who%20did%20not%20microdose%20psychedelics.

Morales-Brown, P. (2024, October 29). What to know about microdosing. https://www.medicalnewstoday.com/articles/microdosing

Roberts, K. (2019, April 19). What to know about microdosing for anxiety and Depression. Allure. https://www.allure.com/story/microdosing-lsd-mushrooms-anxiety-depression

Santos, R., & Santos, R. (2024, August 9). What does microdosing drugs feel like anyway? VICE. https://www.vice.com/en/article/microdosing-drugs-experience-effects-lsd-pscyhedelics/

Syed, O. A., & Tsang, B. (2023). Managing expectations with psychedelic microdosing. Npj Mental Health Research, 2(1). https://doi.org/10.1038/s44184-023-00044-9

Mbs, D. F. L. (2025). Modern Psychedelic Microdosing Research on Mental Health: A Systematic Review. Physicians Postgraduate Press, Inc. https://doi.org/10.4088/pcc.23r03581

www.ingramcontent.com/pod-product-compliance
Lightning Source LLC
LaVergne TN
LVHW012032060526
838201LV00061B/4571